188 Scientific Facts about Teen Sex, Contraception, Pregnancy, Parenting and Sexually Transmitted Infections

Authors: Holly Kreider, Laura Lessard, Denise M. Hill, Diana Dull Akers, and Josefina J. Card

Sociometrics Corporation
170 State Street, Suite 260
Los Altos, CA 94022

Acquisitions Editor: Josefina J. Card
Production Editor: Laurie Rose
Cover Design: Steven Pisano
Composition: Denise M. Hill

ISBN: 978-0-9822492-1-5

Printed in the United States of America by Almaden Press.

SOCIOMETRICS

Foreword

Knowledge is power. This publication is a direct and reliable source of scientific facts on teen sex, contraception, pregnancy, parenting, and sexually transmitted infections. It can be used as supplementary material in sex education classes, as a resource left on a coffee table for teenagers to peruse, and as a stimulus for parent-teen discussions about sex and its consequences. Ultimately, the facts and associated quizzes should help empower youth to make good decisions about their sexual health.

About the Authors

Holly Kreider, Ed.D., is Vice President of Research and Communications and Senior Research Associate at Sociometrics Corporation. She currently leads federally funded and private sector contracts on best-practice adolescent pregnancy prevention, children's mental health, early childhood intervention, parent leadership and family support. She also currently serves on the Board for TeenNOW California (formerly the California Alliance Concerned with School-Age Parenting and Pregnancy Prevention). Prior to joining Sociometrics, Dr. Kreider managed educational research projects and professional development activities at the Harvard Family Research Project (HFRP) for 15 years and served on the faculty at the Harvard Graduate School of Education. She received her Doctorate in Education from Harvard University.

Laura Lessard, M.P.H., is a CDC Foundation Fellow serving in the Coordinating Center for Health Promotion at the Centers for Disease Control and Prevention and a doctoral candidate in the Department of Behavioral Sciences and Health Education at the Rollins School of Public Health, Emory University. She has worked in the public health field as both an evaluator and a researcher for many years, working on diverse topics including HIV/AIDS prevention, teen pregnancy, early childhood health, and most recently obesity prevention. At Sociometrics she served as a Research Associate, collaborating on projects in a number of these areas. Ms. Lessard received her Master of Public Health degree from Tufts University School of Medicine.

Denise M. Hill, B.A., is a former public school teacher and volunteer literacy tutor who obtained both a Multiple Subjects Credential and a Single Subject Credential in English. Later, she spent 11 years at Sociometrics working in office management, operations, and publication design and layout. Currently she is an administrator for the City of Petaluma, as well as a classically trained and certified yoga instructor and certified personal trainer. She received her Bachelor of Arts from California State University, Hayward.

Diana Dull Akers, Ph.D., is a Senior Research Associate at Sociometrics Corporation, where she has led a number of federally funded projects concerning HIV/AIDS prevention and professional development, adolescent reproductive health, alcohol risk reduction and aging. These projects have involved the development and testing of several client-directed, computer-based personal risk assessment and education tools, designed in both English and culturally tailored Spanish formats for use in diverse clinic settings. Dr. Dull Akers previously held a joint teaching appointment in

Sociology and Gender Studies at Sonoma State University. Her areas of interest include social-behavioral approaches to health and illness, gender and sexuality, aging, and ethnographic research methods. She received her PhD in Sociology from the University of California, Santa Cruz.

Josefina J. Card, Ph.D., is Founder and President of Sociometrics Corporation, and a nationally recognized behavioral and social scientist with expertise in the establishment and operation of social science research-based resources, products and services. She has served as Principal Investigator of over 80 R&D projects, many of them multi-year investigations, including the archiving of exemplary datasets and effective prevention programs, and the development of multimedia science-based health educational and training products. Dr. Card has also authored over 80 books, monographs, and journal articles; led training workshops and institutes on science-based prevention program planning, implementation, and evaluation; and served as a member of many federal advisory committees and NIH Study Sections. She received her PhD in Social Psychology from Carnegie-Mellon University.

About Sociometrics

Established in September 1983, Sociometrics Corporation is a research and development firm specializing in health and social/behavioral science research applications. Sociometrics' mission is to produce research-based products and services for diverse audiences, facilitating a fluid and productive feedback loop between science, health practice, and everyday life. This work includes the promotion of evidence-based policymaking; health education of citizens; the replication and dissemination of effective intervention programs for preventing HIV, teen pregnancy, and youth substance abuse; program evaluation research; the facilitation of public access to exemplary behavioral and social data; and the training of non-scientists in the use of social science related technologies and tools.

Table of Contents

chapter 1

teen sex

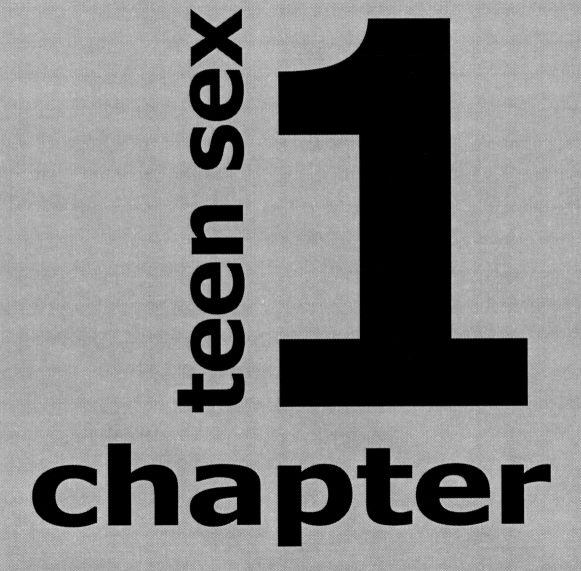

PUBERTY & PEERS

fact 1: reaching sexual maturity

The average age at which women in the U.S. start having their periods (menstruating) is 12.4 years. More than 9 out of every 10 women have had their first period by age 15. [1]

fact 2: early sexual maturity

The past half-century has seen a trend toward earlier sexual maturation for girls in the form of earlier menarche (first period) and onset of breast development. Racial differences are significant, with African-American girls developing earlier than White girls. [62]

fact 3: what do my friends think?

Nine out of ten teens (ages 12-19) agree that it would be easier to delay having sex if their friends or peers spoke positively about not having sex. [2]

fact 4: oral sex only

One in six 15- to 17-year-olds has had oral sex but not sexual intercourse. This percentage varies for racial groups, with 19% of non-Hispanic White, 8% of non-Hispanic Black, and 14% of Hispanic teens ages 15 to 17 reporting having had only oral sex. [3]

fact 5: social norms

Only one-third of teens ages 15 to 19 believe that it is okay for unmarried 16-year-olds to have sex. [1]

fact 6: the birds and the bees

Less than half of young men (33.2%) ever receive information about contraception from their parents or the people who raised them. [1]

fact 7: why wait? age differences

Reasons why teens have never had sex vary by age. Among younger teens, the most frequently cited reason is fear of contracting a sexually transmitted infection. Among older teens, the most frequently cited reason is not having found the right person yet. [1]

fact 8: why wait? ethnic differences

Reasons why teens have never had sex vary by ethnicity. Among non-Hispanic White teens, the most frequently cited reason is that it is against their religion or morals. Among Hispanic teens, the most frequently cited reason is concern about getting (a woman) pregnant. Among non-Hispanic Black teens, the most frequently cited reason is fear of contracting a sexually transmitted infection. [1]

sexual partners

fact 9: looking for true love?

Among teens, the average length of their first sexual relationship was slightly less than six months. [1]

fact 10: steady relationships

Among young women who had sex for the first time between ages 15 to 19, nearly 80% reported that their first experience with sexual intercourse happened with someone they were "going steady" with. [1]

fact 11: pressures to engage in intercourse

Few teens say they didn't really want to have sex the first time (only 6.6% of young men age 15 to 17 and 12% of young women). However, 28.1% of young men ages 15 to 17 who had sex at age 14 or younger reported that they had mixed feelings about having sex the first time. [1]

fact 12: are first partners older?

When young women first have sex, more than 80% of their partners are older. More than 58% of these older partners are 1 to 3 years older. Over 22% are 4 or more years older. [1]

fact 13: casual sex

Young men are more likely to have had sex with a non-romantic partner than young women. In a national survey, about 28% of young men reported having had at least one such sexual experience, compared to 21% of young women. [4]

trends in teen sexual activity: women

fact 14: how many partners?

Among young women ages 15 to 17 in 2005, 12% have had 4 or more partners during their life. The percentages are higher for young Black women than for White and Hispanic young women, with 18.6% of young Black women having had 4 or more partners during their life. [5]

fact 15: oral sex

Half of young women (ages 15 to 19) reported receiving oral sex, but just 44% reported performing oral sex on a partner. [6] Among young women ages 15 to 17, only 36% reported having oral sex (either receiving or performing). [7]

reasons to be cautious: the risks of early sex

fact 16: early sex and number of partners

Young women who have had sexual intercourse earlier in life report greater numbers of sex partners.

The greater the number of sex partners an individual has had, the greater the risk of STI infection. [1]

fact 17: unhealthy relationships

Nine percent of teens reported that their first sexual partner engaged in some form of violence, including pushing and shoving. Twenty-four percent reported that their first sexual partner was verbally abusive. [4]

fact 18: sex and drugs

Almost 30% of sexually active teens (ages 15 to 17) reported that alcohol or drugs has influenced their sexual decision-making; 20% said these situations made them do more than they had planned sexually. [7]

fact 19: communication challenges

Among sexually active teens (ages 15 to 17), 35% of young men and 13% of young women have never had a conversation with their partner about what they feel comfortable doing sexually. Not setting limits by discussing these issues beforehand can make contraceptive use more difficult. [7]

fact 20: on second thought...

Among sexually experienced teens (ages 12-19), 63% wish they had waited longer to have sex. For younger teens (ages 12-14) 81% wish they had waited. [2]

trends in teen sexual activity: men

fact 21: what about the guys?

Among unmarried young men ages 15 to 19, the proportion who had ever had sex declined from 55% in 1995 to 45.7% in 2002. [1] Among 9-12th grade young men responding to an in-school survey, the percentage who had ever had sex was 47.9 in 2005. [5]

fact 22: how many partners?

In 2002, 39% of sexually experienced teen guys reported 2 or more sexual partners in the previous year.

In this same study, 47% of sexually experienced teen guys had only 1 partner in the preceding year, and 7.6% reported 4 or more partners. [1]

fact 23: first sex

In 2002, about 8% of young men said they had had heterosexual intercourse before their 15th birthday, 14.6% by their 16th birthday, 25.3% by their 17th birthday, 39.4% by their 18th birthday, and 54.3% by their 19th birthday.

Young Black men were much more likely to report younger ages at first intercourse than were White young men. For example, the proportion of Black youth who had had intercourse by their 15th birthday was comparable to the levels of first intercourse for young White men by their 17th birthday. [1]

fact 24: one-night stands?

Teen males tend to report higher numbers of one-night stands (e.g. having sex just one time with someone they are not in a relationship with). Twenty-eight percentage of young men reported having one or more one-night stands compared to only 21% of young women. [4]

fact 25: oral sex

Half (52%) of young men reported receiving oral sex while only 39% reported performing oral sex on a partner. [6]

fact 26: multiple partners

Although having sex with multiple partners increases the risk of contracting HIV and other STIs, almost 37% of sexually active 15- to 19-year-old guys reported having four or more sexual partners. This proportion is significantly higher in Black young men, with 46% having four or more partners, as compared to 29% of young White men. [1]

family influences

fact 27: mothers and daughters

A young woman is more likely to have intercourse at an early age if her mother first gave birth as a teen. Among daughters of teen mothers, 56% have had sex by their 20th birthday. In contrast, among other young women, only 41% have had sex by their 20th birthday. [1]

fact 28: religious activity

Teens are less likely to have intercourse before age 18 if their parents attend religious services frequently. Teens who attend religious services themselves are also less likely to have sex before age 18. [8]

fact 29: what do my parents think?

Parent influence is stronger than one might think. A full 37% of teens (age 15 to 19) say that their parents influence their sexual decision-making. Parents themselves underestimated their influence; only 28% said they have influence over their teens' decisions. [9]

fact 30: two parents versus one

Young women who have grown up living with both parents are more likely to delay sexual intercourse than are young women who have grown up in other family situations. Among women who have spent their lives with both parents, 39% have had sex by their 20th birthday. Among other young women, 57% have had sex by their 20th birthday. [1]

fact 31: morals and religious beliefs

Among teens ages 15 to 19 who have never had intercourse, religious beliefs and morals were the most commonly cited reason for delaying sexual activity. Thirty-one percent of young men and 38% of young women said that their religious beliefs and morals were the main reason they have never had intercourse. [1]

fact 32: parents' influence

Teens who reported having a conversation with their parents about how to say no to sex were less likely to report being sexually active. This association was stronger for young men than for women. [1]

fact 33: parents' reaction to 'coming out'

Among gay teens that came out to their parents/guardians, 26% were told they must leave home. [61]

knowledge and behavior

fact 34: survey of high school students

Data from the 2005 Youth Risk Behavior Survey indicate that 87.9% of all high school students in the U.S. had received some form of HIV/AIDS education in school. This percentage has been dropping in recent years, having been as high as 91.5% on 1997. [10]

fact 35: AIDS education

Consistent with the above findings, another national study of young men found that a majority of 15- to 19-year-old young men in the U.S. have received formal instruction about birth control (66%), and resisting sexual activity (83%). Exposure to sex education is associated with modest but significant decreases in the frequency of intercourse in the year prior to the survey. Teens who receive instruction in these topics also show more consistent condom use. [1]

where you

grow UP

makes a difference

fact 36: household type

On average, teens who live in intact families (e.g. live with both biological or adoptive parents) are less likely to report having sex before age 19. [1]

fact 37: state by state

The percentage of teens who report having sex varies by state. Even states that are adjacent to each other have different rates. For example, while 55% of teens in Tennessee report ever having sex, only 46.3% of teens in Kentucky report ever having sex. [5]

fact 38: dad at home

According to a study conducted in the U.S. and New Zealand, young women without fathers at home were twice as likely to have sexual intercourse early and seven times more likely to get pregnant than young women with fathers present. [11]

the transition to being sexually experienced

fact 39: multiple partners

The majority of sexually active 15- to 17-year-olds have had only one sexual partner. [7] [1]

fact 40: effect of sports

Young women who participate in sports are less likely to have sex. When they start having sex, they have sex less often and have fewer partners as compared to non-athletes. [12]

fact 41: having second thoughts about first sex

Nearly one-fourth of teens have sex with their first partner only one time. [4]

fact 42: children of teen moms

Teens whose mother gave birth before turning age 20 are more likely to have sex. Among women with a mother who was a teen parent, 56.3% had had sex by age 19 compared to only 40.6% of young women whose mother was not a teen mom. [1]

fact 43: starting early

In 2005, Black adolescents were significantly more likely to report having first sexual intercourse before age 13 than were White or Hispanic teenagers. Twenty-six percent of Black young men have had sex by age 13 as compared to 5% of White young men and 11% of Hispanic young men. [5]

fact 44: in sheer numbers

In 2002, the estimated number of unmarried 15- to 19-year-old young women who had ever had sexual intercourse was 9.6 million (45.5%). The estimated number of unmarried 15- to 19-year-old men who have ever had sexual intercourse was 10.1 million (45.7%). [1]

fact 45: different rates?

Black young women are more likely to be sexually active as compared to White or Hispanic young women. In 2005, the percentage of young women in high school who had had sex within the past 3 months was 33.5% for White, 43.8% for Black, and 33.7% for Hispanic young women. [5]

fact 46: how often?

Of sexually experienced young women ages 15 to 19, more than 63% have had sex in the last month, more than 92% in the last year. [1]

fact 47: sporadic sex

Among sexually experienced single women who were 15- to 19-years-old in 1995, 3 out of 5 (60%) reported they had sex once a month or less. [1]

fact 48: in sheer numbers

There are approximately 9 million 15- to 19-year-old young men in the U.S. It has been estimated that approximately one-third, or 3 million, are sexually active. [5]

everyone's doing it... or are they?

fact 49: waiting is okay by me

Almost 70% of teens do not think it's okay for high school students to have sex. When asked how many sexual partners teens should have, 56% said, "none." [9]

fact 50: still a virgin by age 17

In 2002, more than 73% of young women were still virgins at age 16, and 57% were still virgins at age 17. [1]

fact 51: ethnic differences?

By their 20th birthdays, Black and Hispanic young men are more likely to have had sex than White young men. [1]

fact 52: sweet 16?

Approximately 14% of teens have had sex by their 16th birthday. In general, Black teens begin to have sex earlier than White teens. According to a national survey, 23% of Black young women and 29% of Black young men have had sex by age 16. Among Whites, 12% and 9% respectively, have done so. [1]

fact 53: which young men have had sex by age 19?

In 1988, 84% of never-married Black men had had sex by age 19, compared with 75% of never-married White men.

In 1995, 85% of never-married Black men had had sex by age 19, compared with 65% of never-married White men.

In 2002, 72.7% of never-married Black men had had sex by age 19, compared with 50.5% of never-married White men. [1]

fact 54: what about the good old days?

Over the 12-year period, 1938 to 1950, an average of 7% of White young women and 51% of White young men had had sex by age 16. At age 20, these figures were 20% for White young women and 73% for White young men. [13]

fact 55: profile

In 2002, the statement "I am an umarried 15- to 19-year old virgin", could be made by: 55% of all young women (55% of White young women, 43% of Black young women, and 63% of Hispanic young women) and 54% of all young men (59% of White young men, 37% of Black young men, and 45% of Hispanic young men). [1]

are you a sexpert?

1. How many 15- to 19-year olds believe it's okay for unmarried 16-year olds to have sex?
A. 1/3
B. 1/4
C. 1/2
D. 3/4

2. More than 75% of young men find out about contraception from parents or guardians. True or False?

3. A teen's relationship with a first sex partner lasts, on average, at least 1 year. True or False?

4. What percentage of sexually active teens report that alcohol or drugs influenced sexual decision making?
a. 15%
b. 20%
c. 30%
d. 42%

5. More than half of young men have had their first heterosexual intercourse experience by age 16. True or False?

6. Teens who reported having a conversation with their parents about how to say no to sex were less likely to report being sexually active. True or False?

7. The percentage of teens in 2005 that have received some sort of HIV/AIDS education is more than 85%. True or False?

8. Young women who participate in sports are less likely to have sex. True or False?

9. In 2002, 57% of young women reported still being virgins at age 17. True or False?

10. Twenty-three percent of Black young women have had sex by age 16 years and 29% of young Black men have had sex by that age. True or False?

rate yourself

Sexpert - 7 to 10 correct
Intermediate - 4 to 6 correct
Novice - 1 to 3 correct

Answers:
1. A. 1/3 (Fact 5); 2. False (Fact 6); 3. False (Fact 9); 4. C. 30% (Fact 18); 5. False (Fact 23); 6. False (Fact 32); 7. True (Fact 39); 8. True (Fact 40); 9. True (Fact 50); 10. True (Fact 52)

2

contraceptive decision making

chapter

contraceptive methods: they're not all alike

fact 56: who uses what?

Sexually active young women under age 20 are more likely to use condoms than other contraceptive methods. Among young women, Blacks are 50% more likely to use injectable contraceptives than Whites (27% vs. 18%); 68% of Whites are using the pill, compared with 55% of Blacks, and 37% of Hispanics. [1]

fact 57: relative to older women

In 2002, American women relied primarily on the more effective methods of contraception, with the pill and condom used by young women and sterilization (female and male) by older women. [1]

barriers to teen contraceptive use

fact 58: parents don't want to talk about it

Sixty-five percent of young women ages 15 to 19 reported that their parents did not talk to them about birth control methods before their 19th birthday. In contrast, only half of young men reported the same. [1]

fact 59: lack of information?

About one in three teens ages 15 to 19 do not receive formal instruction on contraceptive methods before age 18. This lack of formal education may lead to some misperceptions about the effectiveness and side effects of contraception. [1]

fact 60: cost is not an issue

Only 2% of teens stopped using contraception because they could not afford it. [14]

fact 61: side effects

The majority of young women who stopped using contraception did so because of "side effects" including physical side effects (for those using birth control pills) and relationship-related side effects like decreased sexual pleasure and partner dissatisfaction. [14]

fact 62: formal instruction on contraception?

About one-third of both young men and young women report not having received formal instruction on contraceptive methods before age 18. [62]

fact 63: who talks to their parents?

Young women are more likely than young men to talk to their parents about how to say no to sex, methods of birth control, and where to get birth control. [63]

fact 64: young men are less likely to talk to their parents

In 2002, the percentage of young men 18-19 years of age who talked with a parent before age 18 about methods of birth control was 35%. The percentage of young women 18-19 years of age who talked with a parent before age 18 about methods of birth control was 50%. [64]

factors that favor teen contraceptive use

fact 65: just ask!

Research has found that young men whose partners ask them to use a condom are more likely to consistently use one. In addition, young men who say they would feel embarrassed to discuss condoms with a new partner are less likely to consistently use one. [4]

fact 66: does age make a difference?

Regular and effective use of contraception is greater among young women who begin having sexual intercourse in the later, rather than the earlier, teen years. [1]

choosing to use contraceptives

fact 67: choosing the right method

Each contraceptive method has its own set of strengths and challenges and one method might not work for everyone. Between 1995 and 2002, the percentage of sexually active women using injectable contraceptive methods doubled (from 9.7% in 1995 to 20.7% in 2002). Although the percentage of sexually active young women reporting using condoms has remained relatively constant, women are trying other methods to determine what is best for them and their partner. [1]

fact 68: new contraceptive methods

New contraceptive methods don't appear every day, but in recent years, both emergency contraception (also called "Plan B") and the contraceptive patch were introduced. In 2002, 9.6% of sexually active teen women reported ever using one of those two methods. [1]

trends in teen contraception: women

fact 69: users and nonusers of contraception

In 1982, 71% of 15- to 19-year-old sexually active women used contraception at least some of the time. The majority of the contraceptive users—over 6 out of 10—were using the pill. About 2 out of 10 were using condoms.

Twenty years later, in 2002, 83.2% of 15- to 19-year-old sexually active young women used one or more methods at last intercourse. Pill use among teen contraceptors declined to 34.2% and condom use increased significantly to 54.3%. [1]

fact 70: at risk

In 2002, 3.3 million 15- to 19-year-old young women were at risk of an unplanned pregnancy (i.e., they had sex in the last three months). Of these an estimated 2.75 million used contraception. [1]

fact 71: always, sometimes, and never

Among unmarried 15- to 19-year-old sexually active women in 2002, 68% said that they used a condom some or all of the time. Only 21% said they used condoms all of the time. Over 32% said they used condoms none of the time. [1]

fact 72: trying many different methods

In a group of 100 sexually active teen women (age 15 to 19):

- 98 have used a contraceptive method
- 61 have used the pill
- 8 have used emergency contraception
- 94 have used condoms
- 55 have used the withdrawal method [1]

fact 73: race matters

Use of contraception at first intercourse varies by race. Among never-married sexually active teens (ages 15 to 19), the rate of contraception use at first intercourse varied from 71% for Hispanic and non-Hispanic Black women to 78% for non-Hispanic Whites. [1]

fact 74: rate of bisexual or lesbian pregnancy

Overall, bisexual or lesbian respondents were about as likely as heterosexual women ever to have had intercourse (33% and 29%, respectively), but they had a significantly higher prevalence of pregnancy (12%) and physical or sexual abuse (19-22%) than heterosexual or unsure adolescents. [66]

fact 75: being a lesbian or bisexual doesn't preclude becoming pregnant

The majority of adult lesbian and bisexual women have had heterosexual intercourse at some point in their lives, and at least 30% have been pregnant. [67]

trends in teen contraception: men

fact 76: cause for optimism

Among never-married young men (ages 15 to 19) surveyed in 2002, 90.7% used contraception at last intercourse. This compares to only 81.8% in 1995. [1]

fact 77: condom use increases

Among never-married young men (ages 15 to 19), the proportion that used a condom the last time they had sex increased from 63.9% in 1995 to 70.7% in 2002. [1]

fact 78: every time

Although condom use is increasing, only 44% of young men (age 15 to 19) reported using a condom every time they had sex in the past year. This varied considerably by race, with only 29% of non-Hispanic Black young men reporting consistent condom use; compared to 47% of Hispanic young men, and 46% of non-Hispanic White young men. [15]

fact 79: easier said than done

Almost one-third of young men (ages 15 to 19) reported that they feel embarrassed buying condoms at a drugstore. Another 19% thought putting on a condom in front of a partner is embarrassing. [15]

fact 80: decisions, decisions

According to teens (ages 12-17), young women have the most influence over decisions about condoms. The survey found that 49% of teens said young women had the most influence, compared to only 13% who said young men have the most influence. [15]

fact 81: in general

Among sexually experienced young men (ages 15 to 17), 84% report having had a conversation with their partners about using birth control or condoms. [7]

fact 82: under the influence

Almost 7 in 10 teens (ages 15 to 17) agreed with the statement, "People my age often don't use condoms when they are drinking or using drugs." However, only 9% of these teens reported ever having unprotected sex due to alcohol or drug use. [7]

contraceptive use during first intercourse

fact 83: in general

The older a young woman is at first intercourse, the more likely she will be to use c
ception. Among women who were age 14 or younger during their first sexual relatic
26% did not use any method of contraception. Among young women that were ag
older, only 18% did not use any method of contraception. [4]

fact 84: first sex partner

Among teens ages 15 to 19, 21% never used contraception with their first sexual p
Only 63% of teens used contraception every time they had sex with their first
partner. [4]

fact 85: first intercourse and taking contraceptive risks

In 2002, approximately one-fourth of young women who first had sex at ages 15
reported failing to use a contraceptive at first intercourse. Nine in ten reported u
condom. One in ten reported using the "withdrawal method" which is not effec
preventing pregnancy or the spread of STIs, including HIV. [1]

fact 86: relationships make a difference

Teens in romantic relationships with their first sexual partner were more likely to us
traception (80% versus only 64% among those not in romantic relationships). [4]

fact 87: becoming more careful

The proportion of unmarried young men (ages 15 to 19) who were protected by c
ception the first time they had sexual intercourse increased from 73% in 1995 to 8
2002. [1]

fact 88: under the influence

Only 5% of teens reported being under the influence of alcohol or drugs the first tim
had sex. [7]

fact 89: profile

We are 100 never-married young women (ages 15 to 19) typical of those who have already had sex at least once. The first time each of us had sex:

- 17 of us used the pill;
- 68 of us used a condom;
- 8 of us used withdrawal;
- 14 of us used two methods
- Only 25 of us didn't use any contraception at all.

We are 100 never-married young men (ages 15 to 19) typical of those who have already had sex at least once. The first time each of us had sex:

- 15 of us relied on the pill;
- 71 of us used a condom;
- 10 of us used withdrawal;
- 11 of us used two methods
- Only 18 of us didn't use any contraception at all. [1]

contraceptive use at most recent intercourse

fact 90: condoms are gaining in popularity

Among currently sexually active young women in 1995 who used some method of contraception the most recent time they had sex, 45% used hormonal methods (including the pill and Depo-Provera). 54% reported that their partners had used a condom as their means of birth control.

In 2002, 52% used hormonal methods (including the pill and Depo-Provera) and 65% reported using condoms. [1]

fact 91: profile

In 2002, the statement "I am a sexually active, never-married young man between the ages of 15 and 19. I used a condom at last intercourse", could be made by 70.7% of all young men (69.2% of White young men, 86.1% of Black young men). [1]

contraceptive failure

fact 92: good habits

Among young women who did not use birth control at first intercourse, 43% have ever been pregnant. By contrast, among teens that used contraception at first intercourse, only 27% have been pregnant. [16]

are you a sexpert?

1. What method of birth control do sexually active young women under the age of 20 most frequently use?

A. the pill
B. spermicide
C. condoms
D. the patch

2. At least 75% of young women reported that their parents spoke to them about contraceptive methods before the age of 19. True or False?

3. Cost is the major reason teens don't use contraception. True or False?

4. In 2002, nearly 10% of young women reported using either the patch or Plan "B" (emergency contraception). True or False?

5. In 2002, young women used the pill more often than condoms as their method of birth control. True or False?

6. What percentage of young men feel embarrassed about buying condoms?

A. 1/4
B. 1/2
C. 1/3
D. 2/3

7. Which gender has the most influence when it comes to contraception?
A. young women
B. young men

8. Eighty percent of teens used contraception every time they had sex with their first sexual partner. True or False?

9. Twenty-five percent of teens report being under the influence of drugs or alcohol during their first sexual experience. True or False?

10. Condom use as a birth control method increased between 1995 and 2002 among sexually active young women. True or False?

rate yourself

Sexpert - 7 to 10 correct

Intermediate - 4 to 6 correct

Novice - 1 to 3 correct

Answers:
1. C (Fact 56); 2. False (Fact 58); 3. False (Fact 60); 4. True (Fact 68); 5. False (Fact 72); 6. C (Fact 79); 7. A (Fact 80); 8. Fasle (Fact 84); 9. False (Fact 88); 10. True (Fact 90)

fact 98: the facts by state: teen pregnancy

In 2003, the states with the highest number of teen pregnancies were: (1) California with 540,997; (2) Texas with 377,476; (3) New York with 253,714; (4) Florida with 212,250; and (5) Illinois with 182,495.

In 2003, the states with the lowest number of teen pregnancies were: (1) Vermont with 6,589; (2) Wyoming with 6,700; (3) North Dakota with 7,972; (4) Alaska with 10,086; and (5) Delaware with 11,329.

In 2000, the states with the highest teen pregnancy rate (number of pregnancies per 1,000 women age 15 to 19) were: (1) Nevada, 113; (2) Arizona, 104; (3) Mississippi, 103; (4) New Mexico, 103; and (5) Texas, 101.

In 2000, the states with the lowest teen pregnancy rate were: (1) North Dakota with 42; (2) Vermont, 44; (3) New Hampshire, 47; (4) Minnesota, 50; and (5) Maine, 52. [19] [20]

fact 99: the facts by state: teen birth rate

In 2000, the states with the highest teen birth rate (number of births per 1,000 women age 15 to 19) were: (1) Texas, 62.9; (2) New Mexico, 62.7; (3) Mississippi, 62.5; (4) Arizona, 61.1; and (5) Arkansas, 59.0.

In 2000, the states with the lowest teen birth rate were: (1) New Hampshire, 18.2; (2) Vermont, 18.9; (3) Massachusetts, 23.0; (4) Connecticut, 24.8; and (5) Maine, 24.9. [19]

fact 100: outside marriage

In 2003, 97.1% of teen births were to unmarried women. This varied by age. Ninety-five percent (95%) of births among 15-year-old women were to unmarried women. For 16- and 17-year-olds the proportions were 91.1% and 87.7% respectively. [20]

cities where teen pregnancy is most common

fact 101: in absolute numbers

In 2003, of the large U.S. cities, the ones with the most births to teens age 15 to 17 were: (1) New York, New York with 2,868; (2) Washington, DC with 2,577 (3) Los Angeles, California with 2,309; (4) Chicago, Illinois with 2,384; and (5) Houston, Texas with 2,110. [21]

fact 102: birth rates

In 2000, of the 100 largest U.S. cities, the ones with the lowest teen birthrate were Glendale, California (17 births per 1,000 women) and Plano, Texas (20).

The largest cities with the highest teen birthrate were Miami, Florida (174) and Bakersfield, California (121). [22]

the influence of legislation

fact 103: parental notification law

Many states require teens to gain parental permission before obtaining certain types of healthcare services including abortions and other reproductive health services. The medical profession as a whole is against any barriers to teens obtaining care, and statements by the American Medical Association attest to this stance. One research study found that nearly 60% of teens surveyed would stop using reproductive health services and/or delay testing/treatment for STIs if their parents were informed of these actions. [23]

fact 104: access to emergency contraception

Numerous states have passed laws allowing women to obtain emergency contraception (EC) directly from a pharmacist without having to see a physician first. One early study estimated that up to half of the unintended pregnancies that occur each year could be averted if women had access to and used EC. [24]

fact 105: cost of parental consent laws

Parental consent laws often have the effect of forcing teens to delay seeking reproductive healthcare. These delays can amount to an increase in pregnancies, births, abortions and untreated STI's. One study estimated that these laws cost the state of Texas between $11.8 and $56.6 million each year. [25]

international comparisons

fact 106: pregnancy rates

U.S. young women ages 15 to 19 years have a much higher pregnancy rate than young women in European countries. For every 1,000 such women in the U.S. there are nearly 80 pregnancies per year as compared to only 20 in France and only 9 in the Netherlands. [26]

fact 107: abortion rates

There are over 27 abortions per 1,000 women in the U.S. as compared with 10 per 1,000 women in France and 4 per 1,000 in Germany and the Netherlands. [26]

fact 108: comparing the drop in teen births

Although the U.S. saw a dramatic decrease in teen pregnancy during the 1980's and 1990's, this decline was also seen in many countries worldwide. In fact, many countries matched or exceeded the decline in the U.S. (51% decline from 1980 to 1995) including Canada (55% decline), England (56% decline), and Germany (81% decline). [27]

fact 109: differences between american teens and others

As compared to their peers in other countries, teens in the U.S. are more likely to have sex before age 15 and have shorter sexual relationships. Teens in the U.S. are also more likely to have more than one partner in a given year. [28]

from sex to birth

fact 110: attitudes about pregnancy

In one study of young women ages 15 to 19 years, women with an attitude towards pregnancy (either antipregnancy or propregnancy) were more likely to use contraception as compared to those teen women who were ambivalent about pregnancy. In the same study, women who had a positive attitude towards contraception were more likely to use contraception. [29]

fact 111: attitudes towards school

In one study of British teens, women who disliked school were more likely to have unprotected sex and to be pregnant after two years as compared to those who were ambivalent about school. [30]

fact 112: having sex during senior year

In 2005, 49.4% of 12th graders reported having sex at least once in the past three months. [31]

fact 113: use of alcohol and other drugs

Among teens who reported having sex at least once in the past three months, one-fourth reported drinking alcohol or using other drugs the last time they had sex. The percentage varies depending on the age of the teen, with 2.2% of 9th graders and 23.1% of 12th graders reporting drug and/or alcohol use the last time they had sex. [31]

fact 114: so, maybe some teens want to become pregnant?

In a study of young women conducted in California, those teens who were **not** planning on getting pregnant but thought there was a good chance they would get pregnant were more likely to report a pregnancy as compared to young women who thought they had a small chance of getting pregnant. [32]

yes,
i’m pregnant

fact 115: unintended pregnancy

The vast majority of births to teens are unintended. In fact, only 12% of the births to young women age 17 and younger in 2002 were intended. [1]

fact 116: risky business

Women who are Black are more likely than those who are White to be very young the first time they have sex, and also to have sex without contraception. Consequently, Blacks are more likely than Whites to experience a premarital pregnancy, especially at younger ages. [1]

fact 117: alcohol doesn't help

Thirteen percent of teens reported that they've done something sexual while under the influence of alcohol and/or drugs that they might not have done if they were sober. [35]

fact 118: pregnancy and STIs, part one

If a young woman contracts an STI, she is at increased risk for tubal pregnancies and infertility (inability to have babies). [68]

fact 119: pregnancy and STIs, part two

If a pregnant woman contracts an STI, her baby may be at increased risk of having a lung infection, brain infection, eye infection resulting in blindness, birth defect, or being stillborn (born dead). [69]

are you a sexpert?

1. Which group of never-married teens had the highest percentage who reported that they would be upset if they got pregnant or got a partner pregnant?

A. non-Hispanic White young men
B. Hispanic young men
C. non-Hispanic Black young women
D. non-Hispanic White young women

2. If a young woman contracts an STI, she is at increased risk for tubal pregnancies and infertility. True or False?

3. Young women ages 15 to 19 years in European countries have much higher pregnancy rates than those in the U.S. True or False?

4. About one-fourth of teens that reported having sex within the last three months reported drinking alcohol or using drugs the last time they had sex. True or False?

5. The majority of teen pregnancies occur to 15 and 16-year olds. True or False?

6. About 14% of teen pregnancies result in miscarriage. True or False?

7. Approximately one million teen women become pregnant each year. True or False?

8. In 2003, which U.S. city had the most births to teens ages 15 to 17 years?

A. New York, New York
B. Chicago, Illinois
C. Detroit, Michigan
D. Los Angeles, California

9. The majority of teens report that they would stop using reproductive health services and/or delay treatment/testing for STIs if their parents were informed of these actions. True or False?

10. One study estimated that parental consent laws cost the state of Texas between $11.8 and $56.6 million each year. True or False?

rate yourself

Sexpert - 7 to 10 correct

Intermediate - 4 to 6 correct

Novice - 1 to 3 correct

Answers:
1. D (Fact 96); 2. True (Fact 118); 3. False (Fact 106); 4. True (Fact 113); 5. False (Fact 93); 6. True (Fact 97); 7. True (Fact 97); 8. A (Fact 101); 9. True (Fact 103); 10. True (Fact 105)

chapter 4

teen parenting

head count of babies born to teens

fact 120: every three minutes

A teen gives birth. [1]

fact 121: every day

Close to 500 babies are born every day in the U.S. to women ages 17 and younger. [1]

fact 122: over time

The birthrate (number of births per 1,000 women) for 15- to 19-year-olds decreased from 62 in 1991 to 41.9 in 2006. The rate decreased for Whites (dropping from 43.4 to 26.6), Hispanics (dropping from 104.6 to 83), as well as for Blacks (from 118.2 to 63.7). [33]

fact 123: a decline in teen birth rates during the '90s

During the 1990s, there was a steady decline in the teenage birthrate (number of births per 1,000 women). Black teens experienced the most substantial decrease, declining from 118.2 in 1991 to 60.9 in 2005—a drop of almost 48%. The birthrate for the other ethnic groups also decreased between 22 and 40 percent during that time. [33]

fact 124: a recent up tick in teen birth rates

While the birthrate for teenagers declined notably from 68.3 (per 1,000 women) in 1970 to 40.5 in 2005, preliminary estimates for the 2006 birthrate showed a 3% increase to 41.9 per 1,000 women.

According to the National Campaign to Prevent Teen Pregnancy, there are four plausible explanations for this increase:

- Complacency among policy makers and funders of teen pregnancy prevention programs.
- Since the birth rate for all ages has increased, there may be other factors impacting the birth rate of all women (i.e., the up tick is not a specific issue among teens).
- The current generation of teen women need different prevention programs and services than previous generations; the current system is not working for today's teens.

- The increase in all unmarried births (including births to older women) may be related to the increase in births to teens, since the majority (60%) of teen moms are not married. [33, 60]

fact 125: in sheer numbers

In 2006 there were approximately 441,833 births to U.S. teens:

- 141,107 births among non-Hispanic White young women
- 106,162 births among non-Hispanic Black young women
- 8,344 births among American Indian or Alaska Native young women
- 7,743 births among Asian or Pacific Islander young women
- 148,106 births among Hispanic young women [33]

fact 126: probability of a first birth

1% by age 15
2% by age 16
4% by age 17
9% by age 18
13% by age 19
18% by age 20 [1]

fact 127: racial and ethnic differences

Teen birthrates vary substantially by race and ethnicity. In 2006, among young women ages 15 to 19, the numbers of births per 1,000 women were: 16.7 among Asians and Pacific Islanders, 26.6 among non-Hispanic Whites, 54.7 among American Indians, 83.0 among Hispanics, and 63.7 among non-Hispanic Blacks. [33]

fact 128: older vs. younger teens

A higher percentage of older teen women become mothers each year than younger women. In 2006, the birth rate among teens ages 18- to 19-years-old was 73 (per 1,000 women). Among 15- to 17-year-olds, the birth rate was 22 and among 10- to 14-year-olds the birth rate was just 0.6. [33]

fact 129: first-time mothers

In 2006, the birthrate for young women ages 15 to 19 having a first child was 33.7 per 1,000 women. Among young women having a second, third or fourth child, the birth rate was 8.2 per 1,000 women. [33]

fact 130: repeat births

In 2004, one-fifth of births to younger women ages 15 to 19 were repeat births. This means that nearly 83,000 births were to teen mothers who had already given birth. The percentage of births that are repeat births varies by state from 12% of teen births in Vermont to 24% of births in Texas. [34]

adoption

fact 131: choosing adoption

The number of single teen mothers ages 15- to 19-years old choosing to place their babies for adoption declined dramatically over the past 30 years. Between 1982 and 1988, 3% of White teens placed their child for adoption. Current research shows that only 1% of teen parents place their child for adoption. [37] [38]

fact 132: father's opinion counts

One study found that the most powerful predictor of young women's decision to give their child up for adoption was the birth fathers' preference. [39]

fact 133: family support for adoption

According to teens surveyed by one research team, adolescents who decide to place their baby for adoption most often come from upper-middle-class families and from intact families with highly educated parents. The teens in this study reported that their decision to give their baby up for adoption was highly influenced by their friends and siblings and by knowing someone who was adopted or being adopted themselves. [39]

fact 134: teens can make their own adoption choices

In 40 states and the District of Columbia, a mother who is a minor may legally place her child for adoption without her parent's involvement. [70]

abortion

fact 135: teen abortion trends

In 1972, over 32% of abortions were obtained by women age 19 and younger. In 2004, that percentage dropped to only 17.4% of all abortions. [40, 41]

fact 136: latest figures

Although teenagers' abortion rate has declined relative to women of other ages since 1987, the abortion rate has increased among women in their early 20s. [40, 41]

fact 137: how prevalent?

In 2004, there were just under 800 legally induced abortions for every 1,000 live births to young women up to age 15. For young women age 15 to 19, there were just under 400 abortions for every 1,000 live births. [41]

fact 138: state by state

New York, Ohio and Pennsylvania have some of the highest numbers of abortions to young women up to age 15. In New York City, over 550 abortions were performed to teens younger than 15.

Of teens ages 15 to 19, the most abortions were performed in New York, Texas and Illinois. [41]

fact 139: family support

An analysis of a national dataset found that family factors including whether or not the family pays attention to the young woman or understands the young woman were not associated with a young woman's decision to abort a pregnancy. The study did find that teens who responded "not at all" or "very little" when asked if they would like to leave home were significantly less likely to abort a pregnancy. [42]

fact 140: teen abortion

In 2004, about one in six legally-induced abortions were obtained by women under the age of 20. [41]

fact 141: psychological consequences

Young women who decide to abort a pregnancy are more likely to report receiving counseling for psychological or emotional problems and are more likely to report trouble sleeping over the past year as compared to young women that give birth. [42]

for whom the teen wedding bells ring

fact 142: are more teens marrying these days?

In 1988, the percentage of 15- to 19-year-old young women who were ever married was 3%; by 2006 this figure had dropped to 2.4%.

In 1988, the percentage of 15- to 19-year-old young men who were ever married was under 1%; by 2006 this figure had increased to 1.4%. [43]

fact 143: hispanics are most likely to be married as teens

In 2006, 4.6% of 15- to 19-year-old Hispanic young women were married. For White young women and Black young women, these figures were (only) 2.1% and 1.7%, respectively. [43]

fact 144: younger teen moms are rarely married

About 11.5% of teen mothers age 17 and younger are married as compared to 32.1% of mothers age 18-19 and 48.6% of mothers age 20-21. [44]

fact 145: over time

There have been marked changes in married and unmarried childbearing among U.S. teenagers 15- to 19-years-of-age:

The birth rate for married younger women decreased from 420.2 births per 1,000 married women in 1990 to 283.6 in 2002.

The birth rate for unmarried younger women decreased from 45.8 births per 1,000 unmarried women in 1994 to 34.5 in 2005. [45]

fact 146: less likely to marry the birth mother

Eight of ten teen fathers do not marry the mothers of their first children. These absent fathers pay less than $800 annually for child support, often because they are quite poor themselves. [71]

parenting without marriage

fact 147: going it alone

The majority of teen births in the U.S. are taking place out-of-wedlock. In 2006, only 16% of births to teens occurred to married young women. [45]

fact 148: it's not only teens that are opting not to marry

In 2005, 37% of all births in the U.S. occurred outside marriage. Experts believe this is partially due to the high number of couples who live together, but are not married, deciding to have children. [46]

fact 149: increases and decreases

Not surprisingly, married teens are much more likely to have children than unmarried teens. In 2002, there were 284 births per 1,000 married women ages 15- to 19-years old, compared to 35 births per 1,000 unmarried women in the same age range. [45]

education

fact 150: achieving future goals

A national study of men and women ages 12 to 19 found that teens believe becoming a teen parent would negatively impact their future. Forty percent (40%) of teens surveyed said it would, "prevent [them] from reaching [their] goals for the future" and another 41% reported that it would, "delay [them] from reaching [their] goals for the future". Only 10% said it wouldn't affect their ability to reach their goals. [47]

fact 151: high school diplomas

According to a national survey, only 40% of young teen mothers (ages 17 or younger) receive a high school diploma. Less than 2% of these moms complete a college degree by age 30. [48]

fact 152: what about the g.e.d. (general educational development)?

Many teen mothers obtain a General Educational Development (G.E.D.) certificate. If the GED is considered the equivalent of a high school diploma, the educational gap between teen mothers and women who delay childbearing is reduced even further. Researchers debate whether a GED has the same value as a high school diploma for women in the labor market.

fact 153: what about college?

By the age of 30, only 5% of young teen mothers and 10% of older teen mothers complete at least two years of college, and less than 2% of young teen mothers and 3% of older teen mothers obtain a college degree. Comparatively, 21% of women who delay childbirth complete at least two years of college, and 9% graduate. [72]

fact 154: less school for teen dads

Teen fathers are more likely to engage in delinquent behaviors such as alcohol and drug abuse or drug dealing, and they complete fewer years of schooling than their childless peers. [73]

children of teen parents

fact 155: low birth weight

Children born to very young mothers have a greater risk of being born with a low birth weight (under 2,500 grams, or 5 pounds 8 ounces). In one study, children born to teens age 17 and younger were significantly more likely to be born with low birth weight as compared to children of mothers age 20-29. The risk can be offset by adequate prenatal care. [44]

fact 156: at risk...

Children born to teen mothers are at greater risk of experiencing problems with health and cognitive development. On average these children have significantly lower fine motor skills and composite motor skills as compared to children with mothers ages 25-29. [44]

fact 157: profile

"I was born with a low birth weight (i.e. under 2,500 grams, or 5 pounds 8 ounces)." This statement can be made by:

7.2% of babies born to mothers younger than 17 years old
5.2% of babies born to 18- and 19-year-old mothers
2.7% of babies born to 20- and 21-year-old mothers
4.2% of babies born to 22- through 24-year-old mothers
4.3% of babies born to 25- through 29-year-old mothers [44]

fact 158: lasting effects

Teen mothers may provide less cognitive stimulation to their children than women who delay childbearing. Children of teen mothers tend to show poorer cognitive development and have significantly lower test scores in reading, math and general knowledge then children of older mothers ages 25-29. [44]

fathers: effects on teen dads

fact 159: do fathers influence pregnancy intentions?

Although the majority of teenage pregnancies are unplanned and unwanted, one study of African-American teen fathers found that nearly 40% of the births were wanted by the fathers. In addition, the majority of fathers supported the idea of teen parenting. [49]

fact 160: parenting stress

Using data from 50 mother-father teen parent dads, researchers determined that teen fathers with less contact with their child were more likely to suffer from parenting stress as compared to fathers who were more involved with their children. The study also found that whether or not a father lives with the child is not strongly associated with the father's involvement in the child's life. This means that even if a teen father does not live with the mother or child, he can still be highly involved in the life of the child. [50]

fact 161: he said, she said

According to teen fathers, the most common reasons for decreasing involvement in the child's life are degrading relationships with the mother or maternal grandparents, or financial concerns. According to teen mothers, the most common reason is disinterest on the part of the father. [36]

fact 162: expectations

One study found that teen fathers receive considerably less support as compared to teen mothers. This includes less support from their families and limited or no contact with social workers and medical professionals. [36]

cost to society

fact 163: decades of teen parents

Between 1991 and 2004, 6,776,230 children were born to teens in the U.S.. The public costs for teen childbearing over this period was over $160 billion dollars. [48]

fact 164: starting young

Taxpayers shell out $4,080 per year per person for teen mothers ages 17 and younger. [48]

fact 165: annual costs

According to one estimate, U.S. taxpayers spent over $9 billion on teen childbearing-related costs in 2004.

These costs include:
$1.9 billion for health care costs
$2.3 billion for child welfare
$2.1 billion for state prison systems
$2.9 billion in lost tax revenue due to teen mothers making less money over their lifetime [48]

earning power

fact 166: teen mothers earn less

Teen mothers earn on average $6,900 per year between the ages of 18 and 35. This is $3,350 per year less than those who delay their first birth until age 20 or 21. [48]

fact 167: teen parenthood and poverty

Teen mothers are more likely to suffer from poverty in their teen and adult years than are their friends, neighbors, and classmates who delay childbearing until their 20s and 30s. [48]

fact 168: teen moms and child neglect and abuse

Children born to teenage mothers are more likely have a child neglect/abuse report by age 5. Children of teen mothers are also more likely to be placed in foster care. The researchers estimated that delaying the age at first birth nationally from 17 years and under to 18-19 years would save U.S. taxpayers about $150 million in foster care expenses. [51]

are you a sexpert?

1. Every 15 minutes a teen gives birth. True or False?

2. What happened to the teen birth rate in the 1990s from the prior decade?

A. it doubled
B. it tripled
C. it didn't change significantly
D. it steadily declined

3. Which group of teens had the highest number of births in 2006?

A. Hispanic teen women
B. Non-Hispanic Black teen women
C. Non-Hispanic White teen women
D. Asian teen women

4. What percentage of births to teen women ages 15-19 are repeat births?

A. 50%
B. 33%
C. 25%
D. 20%

5. The most powerful predictor of teen women's decisions to place their child for adoption is the birth father's preference. True or False?

6. Over the last 30 years, the number of single teen mothers ages 15-19 choosing to place their babies for adoption has:

A. declined slightly
B. declined dramatically
C. risen slightly
D. risen dramatically

7. New York, Florida and California are the three states with the highest number of abortions among teens 15 and younger. True or False?

8. Which group is mostly likely to be married as teens?

A. Non-Hispanic Whites
B. Asians
C. Hispanics
D. Non-Hispanic Blacks

9. As of 2006, 31% of births to teens occurred among teens that were married. True or False?

10. Which of the following statements is true regarding children of teen parents?

A. they are at greater risk of being low-birth weight babies
B. they tend to have significantly lower fine motor skills
C. they tend to have poorer cognitive development
D. all of the above

rate yourself

Sexpert - 7 to 10 correct
Intermediate - 4 to 6 correct
Novice - 1 to 3 correct

Answers:
1. False (Fact 120); 2. D (Fact 123); 3. A (Fact 125); 4. D (Fact 130); 5. True (Fact 132); 6. B (Fact 131); 7. False (Fact 138); 8. C (Fact 143); 9. False (Fact 147); 10. D (Fact 155, 156, 158)

chapter 5

teen sexually transmitted infections

sex can do more than get teens pregnant: STIs

fact 169: sexually transmitted infections (STIs): the big picture

The Centers for Disease Control and Prevention has estimated that nearly 19 million new cases of STIs occur in the U.S. each year, 9 million (48%) to teenagers. Adolescents and young adults ages 20-24 are at higher risk for sexually transmitted infection than are older individuals. In addition, one in three sexually active young adults becomes infected with an STI before age 24. [52, 53]

fact 170: gonorrhea

As in previous years, in 2006 women ages 15 to 19 had the highest rate of gonorrhea diagnoses as compared to any other age/sex group. There were 647.9 cases per 100,000 population meaning that over 6 in every 1,000 women ages 15 to 19 was diagnosed with gonorrhea during that year. [54]

fact 171: chlamydia

Gonorrhea and chlamydia are the most common STIs among teens. Young women ages 15 to 19 had the highest gonorrhea rate of any age group of women in 2006. Young men (ages 15 to 19) had the second highest rate, faring better than 20-24 year old men.

Chlamydia rates have increased since 2002. The rates are consistently higher for women than for men. In 2006, the rate of chlamydia among 15- to 19-year-old young men was 545.1 per 100,000 and for young women the rate was 2,862.7 per 100,000. [54]

fact 172: not just the women

Between 2002 and 2004, gonorrhea cases decreased every year among 15- to 19-year-old guys. This trend has changed, however, and between 2005 and 2006, the rate of reported cases of gonorrhea increased 8.4%.

2002: 285.7 per 100,000

2003: 261.2 per 100,000

2004: 250.2 per 100,000

2005: 257.5 per 100,000

2006: 279.1 per 100,000 [54]

fact 173: herpes virus

Although few teens with the herpes virus have visible symptoms, it remains a common STI among teens. Contracting herpes (or any other STI) increases the risk of HIV transmission. [55]

fact 174: syphilis

Syphilis remains relatively uncommon among teens, with only 565 reported cases among 15- to 19-year olds in 2006 (a rate of 2.7 per 100,000). [54]

fact 175: hiv/aids

Relatively few teens have AIDS. However, there were more than 4,000 teens ages 15 to 19 living with HIV in 2005. [56]

fact 176: hpv

Over 4.6 million new cases of human papillomavirus (HPV) are diagnosed every year among persons age 15 to 24. This virus causes genital warts and has been linked to the development of cervical cancer. A vaccine for certain strains of HPV (HPV 6,11, 16 and 18) has been approved and is recommended to women ages 9-26 years. [52]

fact 177: sti transmission routes

There are two primary ways that STIs are transmitted. Some STIs (such as HIV, chlamydia, and gonorrhea) are transmitted when secretions from the urethra or vagina come in contact with mucosal surfaces (such as genital herpes, syphilis). Other STIs, such as human papillomavirus are primarily transmitted through contact with skin or mucosal surfaces. [74]

common STIs and their symptoms

fact 178: symptoms of the most common STIs in teens

Chlamydia:
- Genital discharge
- Burning when urinating
- If left untreated, it can lead to pelvic inflammatory disease

Gonorrhea:
- Discharge from the genital organs
- Burning or itching during urination

HPV:
- Genital warts (sometimes warts are not visible)
- Most people with HPV have no symptoms

Herpes:
- Itching, burning, or pain in the genital area
- Blisters or sores (sores heal but may re-appear)
- Fever, headaches and/or other muscle aches

Syphilis:
- Painless sores on genitals (10 days to 3 months after infection)
- Swollen lymph glands [57]

health consequences of STIs

fact 179: consequences of STIs

Some curable STIs (like gonorrhea or chlamydia) can cause serious health problems if not diagnosed and treated early:

- Pelvic inflammatory disease (PID)
- Tubal pregnancy (also called ectopic pregnancy)
- Infertility

Infection with genital warts (human pappillomavirus or HPV) has been linked to certain types of cancers later on.

AIDS is caused by infection with human immunodeficiency virus (HIV). People who develop AIDS suffer from severely weakened immune systems, which leave them susceptible to infections. There is no cure for AIDS at this time. [57]

fact 180: syphilis: new life for an old infection

If not treated, syphilis can cause blindness, heart disease, mental illness, joint damage, and death.

Pregnant women who are infected can transmit the infection to their unborn children, who often die before birth or soon afterward. [57]

fact 181: which STIs can be cured? which ones can't?

STIs caused by bacteria (like chlamydia, gonorrhea, and syphilis) can usually be cured with antibiotics if diagnosed early. However, because these infections often produce mild or no symptoms early on—especially in women—they may not be treated until serious problems develop.

STIs caused by viruses—genital herpes, genital warts, and AIDS—cannot be cured, although some medications may reduce the severity and/or delay the appearance of symptoms. [57]

fact 182: annual screening

Chlamydia is an STI with potentially serious long-term consequences, including pelvic inflammatory disease (PID) and infertility. The CDC recommends annual chlamydia screening of all sexually active women ages 25 and under. [75]

pregnancy prevention does not always equal STI prevention

fact 183: how safe is doing everything but "going all the way"?

Although remaining a virgin (not ever having sexual intercourse) eliminates the possibility of becoming pregnant, it may not prevent the transmission of STIs. Sexual activities other than intercourse, such as oral sex and anal sex, can spread STIs. Oral sex can transmit oral, respiratory and genital pathogens including STIs such as herpes, hepatitis, gonorrhea, chlamydia, syphilis and even HIV. [58]

fact 184: oral sex and transmission

Although oral sex can transmit various infections including chlamydia, in one study, 14% of teens surveyed incorrectly thought the risk of contracting chlamydia through oral sex was absolutely zero. [58]

fact 185: a note about condoms

Condoms provide different levels of protection for various STIs, depending on how they are transmitted. Condoms provide less protection for genital ulcer type infections (e.g. herpes, syphilis, HPV) because these infections also may be transmitted by exposure to areas not covered or protected by the condom. [76]

preventing STIs

fact 186: preventing STIs and pregnancy

Correct and consistent use of a latex condom (or polyurethane condom for those with latex allergies) at each intercourse significantly reduces the chances of becoming infected with an STI, including HIV. Incorrect or inconsistent condom use may be just as harmful as no use at all. In one study, more than one-fourth of teens using condoms inconsistently and/or incorrectly tested positive for an STI compared to 7% of those reporting consistent and correct use. [59]

fact 187: using the right lube

Petroleum- or oil-based lubricants (such as petroleum jelly, body oils or lotions, cooking oils or shortening, etc.) can weaken latex condoms, increasing STI risks. Only water-based lubricants should be used with condoms. [77]

fact 188: the truth about hiv transmission

Human immunodeficiency virus (HIV), the virus that causes AIDS, cannot be transmitted through air, water, insects or casual contact. HIV is transmitted in one of three ways: 1) by sexual contact (anal, vaginal, or oral) with someone infected with HIV; 2) by sharing needles and/or syringes with someone infected with HIV; 3) babies born to HIV-infected women may become infected before or during birth or through breast feedings. [78]

are you a sexpert?

1. Herpes and syphilis are the most common STIs among teens. True or False?

2. Which statement is true regarding young men and gonorrhea?

A. men don't get gonorrhea, only women do.
B. in 2001 a vaccine was created that can treat male gonorrhea.
C. gonorrhea cases among young men declined for years, but rose in 2005.
D. gonorrhea cases for young men have been going up for the past 20 years.

3. Herpes increases teens' risk for HIV. True or False?

4. Which STI is relatively uncommon among teens?

A. gonorrhea
B. syphilis
C. herpes
D. HPV

5. Which of the following STIs has a vaccine, recommended for girls and women ages 9-26?

A. HIV
B. HPV
C. herpes
D. chlamydia

6. Which serious health problems can occur if certain STIs are not treated early?

A. infertility
B. tubal pregnancies
C. pelvic inflammatory disease
D. all of the above

7. Which STIs can be cured if treated early?

A. STIs caused by bacteria
B. STIs caused by viruses
C. STIs caused by both bacteria and viruses
D. to date, there are no cures for any STIs

8. Which types of sexual activity present no risk for STI infection?

A. oral sex
B. anal sex
C. vaginal sex
D. none of the above

9. Correct and consistent use of condoms reduces the chances you will get pregnant or get an STI. True or False?

10. To minimize STI transmission risk, which of the following sexual lubricants is safest to use with condoms?

A. baby oil
B. vaseline
C. water-based lubricants
D. body lotion

rate yourself

Sexpert - 7 to 10 correct

Intermediate - 4 to 6 correct

Novice - 1 to 3 correct

Answers:
1. False (Fact 174); 2. C (Fact 172); 3. True (Fact 173); 4. B (Fact 174); 5. B (Fact 176); 6. D (Fact 179); 7. A (Fact 181); 8. D (Fact 183); 9. True (Fact 186); 10. C (Fact 187)

references

1. Abma, J., Martinez, G.M., Mosher, W.D., & Dawson, B.S. (2004). Teenagers in the U.S.: Sexual activity, contraceptive use, and childbearing, 2002. Washington DC: National Center for Health Statistics, Series 23: Data from the National Survey of Family Growth, (24), 1-48.

2. The National Campaign to Prevent Teen Pregnancy. (2003). Science Says: The Case for the Cautious Generation. (Issue No. 2). Washington, DC: Author. Retrieved 11/26/2007 from http://www.thenationalcampaign.org/resources/pdf/SS/SS2_CautiousGen.pdf

3. Terry-Humen, E., Manlove, J. & Cottingham, S. (2006). Trends and recent estimates: Sexual activity among U.S. teens. (Publication No. 2006-08). Washington, DC: Child Trends Research Briefs.

4. Ryan, S., Manlove, J. & Franzetta, K. (2003). The first time: Characteristics of teens' first sexual relationships. (Publication No. 2003-16). Washington, DC: Child Trends Research Briefs.

5. Eaton, D.K., Kann, L., Kinchen, S., Ross, J., Hawkins, J., Harris, W.A., Lowry, R., McManus, T., Chyen, D., Shanklin, S., Lim, C., Grunbaum, J. A., Wechsler, H. (2006). Youth Risk Behavior Surveillance - U.S., 2005. MMWR Surveill Summ. 55(5), 1-108.

6. The National Campaign to Prevent Teen Pregnancy. (2005). Science says: Teens and oral sex. (Issue No. 17). Washington, DC: Author. Retrieved 11/26/2007 from http://www.thenationalcampaign.org/resources/pdf/SS/SS17_OralSex.pdf

7. Hoff, T., Greene, L., & Davis, J. (2003). National survey of adolescents and young adults: Sexual health knowledge, attitudes and experiences. Menlo Park, CA: The Henry J. Kaiser Family Foundation. Retrieved 11/26/2007 from http://www.kff.org/youthhivstds/upload/National-Survey-of-Adolescents-and-Young-Adults-Sexual-Health-Knowledge-Attitudes-and-Experiences-Summary-of-Findings.pdf

8. The National Campaign to Prevent Teen Pregnancy. (2005).Science Says: The association between parent, family and peer religiosity and teenagers' sexual experience and contraceptive use. (Issue No. 20). Washington, DC: Author. Retrieved 11/26/2007 from http://www.thenationalcampaign.org/resources/default.aspx

9. Albert, B. (2003). With one voice 2004: America's adults and teens sound off about teen pregnancy. Washington, DC: The National Campaign to Prevent Teen Pregnancy. Retrieved 11/26/2007 from http://www.thenationalcampaign.org/resources/pdf/pubs/WOV_2004.pdf

10. Youth Risk Behavior Survey. (2007). Trends in the Prevalence of Sexual Behaviors. Washington, DC: Centers for Disease Control and Prevention. Retrieved 12/11/2007 from http://www.cdc.gov/HealthyYouth/yrbs/pdf/yrbs07_us_sexual_behaviors_trend.pdf

11. Ellis, B.J., Bates, J.E., Dodge, K.A., Fergusson, D.M., & Horwood, L.J. (2003). Does father absence place daughters at special risk for early sexual activity and teenage pregnancy. Child Development, 74, 801-82.

12. The National Campaign to Prevent Teen Pregnancy (2003). Not just another single issue: Teen pregnancy and athletic involvement. Washington, DC: Author. Retrieved 12/28/2007 from http://www.thenationalcampaign.org/resources/default.aspx

13. Moore, K. A., Wenk, D., Hofferth, S. L., & Hayes, C. D. (1987). Statistical appendix: Trends in adolescent sexual and fertility behavior., in S. Hofferth & C. Hayes (Eds.), Risking the future: Adolescent sexuality, pregnancy, and childbearing (pp. 353-503). Washington DC: National Academy Press.

14. The National Campaign to Prevent Teen Pregnancy. (2006). Science says: Teen contraceptive use. (Issue No. 29). Washington, DC: Author. Retrieved July 7, 2009 from http://www.thenationalcampaign.org/resources/pdf/SS/SS29_Contraceptive.pdf

15. The National Campaign to Prevent Teen Pregnancy. (2003). Science says: The sexual attitudes and behavior of male teens. (Issue No. 6). Washington, DC: Author. Retrieved 11/26/2007 from http://www.thenationalcampaign.org/resources/pdf/SS/SS6_MaleTeens.pdf

16. The National Campaign to Prevent Teen Pregnancy. (2006). Science says: Pregnancy among sexually experiences teens, 2002. (Issue No. 23). Washington, DC: Author. Retrieved 11/26/2007 from http://www.thenationalcampaign.org/resources/pdf/SS/SS23_ExpTeens.pdf

17. Guttmacher Institute. (2006). Facts of American teen's sexual and reproductive health. Washington, DC: Author. Retrieved on 11/26/2007 from http://www.guttmacher.org/pubs/fb_ATSRH.pdf

18. The National Campaign to Prevent Teen Pregnancy. (2006). Science says: Teens' attitudes toward pregnancy and childbearing, 1988-2002. (Issue No. 21). Washington, DC: Author. Retrieved 11/26/2007 from http://www.thenationalcampaign.org/resources/pdf/SS/SS21_TeensAttitudes.pdf

19. The National Campaign to Prevent Teen Pregnancy. (2005). Teen pregnancy and birth rates in the U.S. Washington, DC: Author. Retrieved November 26, 2007, from: http://www.thenationalcampaign.org/resources/default.aspx

20. Martin, J. A., Hamilton, B. E., & Sutton, P. D. (2005). Births: Final data for 2003. National Vital Statistics Report, 54(2). Hyattsville, MD: National Center for Health Statistics.

21. Child Trends. (2004). Fast facts at a glance. Washington, DC: Author. Retrieved November 26, 2007, from: http://www.childtrends.org/_listES.cfm?LID=C33B0F7B-0ACC-41C4-A7E8C8B675B22EF6.

22. Annie E. Casey Foundation. (2003). Teen births in America's largest cities: 1990 and 2000. Baltimore, MD: Author.

23. Eisenberg, M., Swain, C., Bearinger, L.H. & Sieving, R.E. (2005). Parental notification laws for minors' access to contraception: What do parents say? Archives of Pediatric and Adolescent Medicine, 159 (2), 120-125.

24. Raine, T., Harper, C.C., Rocha, C.H., Fisher, R., Padian, N., Klausner, J.D., & Darney, P.D. (2005). Direct access to emergency contraception through pharmacies and effect on unintended pregnancy and STIs. JAMA, 293 (1), 54-62.

25. Franzini, L.,Marks, E., Cromwell, P.F., Risser, J., McGill, L., Markham, C., Selwyn, B., & Shapiro, C. (2004). Projected economic costs due to health consequences of teenagers' loss of confidentiality in obtaining reproductive health care services in Texas. Archives of Pediatric and Adolescent Medicine,158, 1140-1146.

26. Advocates for Youth (2003). Adolescent sexual health in Europe and the U.S. - What's the difference? Washington, DC: Author.

27. Lawlor, D. & Shaw, M. (2004). Teenage pregnancy rates: high compared with where and when? Journal of the Royal Society of Medicine, 97(3), 121-123.

28. Singh, S. & Darroch, J. (1999). Adolescent pregnancy and childbearing: Levels and trends in developed countries. Family Planning Perspectives, 32 (1).

29. Bruckner, H., Martin, A. & Bearman, P. (2004). Ambivalence and pregnancy: Adolescents' attitudes, contraceptive use and pregnancy. Perspectives on Sexual and Reproductive Health, 36(6), 248-257.

30. Bonnell, C., Allen, E., Strange, V., Copas, A., Oakley, A., Stephenson, J., & Johnson, A. (2005). The effect of dislike of school on risk of teenage pregnancy: Testing of hypotheses using longitudinal data from a randomized trial of sex education. Journal of Epidemiology and Community Health, 59, 223-230.

31. National Center for Chronic Disease Prevention and Health Promotion. (2007). Youth online: Comprehensive results (YRBSS data). Washington, DC: Centers for Disease Control and Prevention.

32. Rosengard, C., Phipps, M. & Adler, N. (2004). Adolescent pregnancy intentions and pregnancy outcomes: a longitudinal examination. Journal of Adolescent Health, 35(6), 453-461.

33. Hamilton, B., J. Martin, & Ventura, S. (2007). Births: Preliminary data for 2006. National Vital Statistics Reports, 56(7). Hyattsville, MD: National Center for Health Statistics.

34. Schelar, E., Franzetta, K. & Manlove, J. (2005). Repeat teen childbearing: Differences across states and by race and ethnicity. Research Briefs. Washington DC: Child Trends.

35. The National Campaign to Prevent Teen Pregnancy. (2005). Sobering facts on alcohol and teen pregnancy. Washington, DC: Author. Retrieved December 28, 2007, from: http://www.thenationalcampaign.org/resources/default.aspx

36. Bunting, L. & McAuley, C. (2004). Teenage pregnancy and parenthood: the role of fathers. Child & Family Social Work, 9 (3), 295-303.

37. Terry, N., Turner, N. & Falkner, J. (2005). Current issues with child adoption. Paper presented at the Allied Academies International Internet Conference, Las Vegas, CA.

38. Alan Guttmacher Institute. (1994). Sex and America's teenagers. New York. NY: Author.

39. Child Welfare Information Gateway. (2005). Voluntary relinquishment for adoption. Washington, DC: Author. Retrieved 12/28/2007, from http://www.childwelfare.gov/pubs/s_place.cfm

40. Elam-Evans, L. D., Strauss, L. T., Herndon, J., Parker, W. Y., Bowens, S. V., Zane, S., Berg, C. J. (2002). Abortion surveillance - U.S., 1999. MMWR Surveill Summ, 51(9), 1-28.

41. Strauss, L., Gamble, S. B., Parker, W. Y., Cook, D. A., Zane, S. B., & Hamdan, S. (2006). Abortion surveillance - U.S., 2004. MMWR Surveill Summ, 56(9), 1-33.

42. Coleman, P. (2006). Resolution of unwanted pregnancy during adolescence through abortion versus childbirth: individual and family predictors and psychological consequences. Journal of Youth and Adolescence,35, 903-911.

43. U.S. Census Bureau. (2006). 2006 American community survey. Washington, DC: U.S. Government Printing Office.

44. Terry-Humen, E., Manlove, J. & Moore, K. (2005). Playing catch-up: how children born to teen mothers fare. Washington DC: National Campaign to Prevent Teen Pregnancy.

45. Child Trends Data Bank. (2007). Teen Births. Washington, DC: Author. Retrieved month, date, year, from: http://www.childtrendsdatabank.org/indicators/13TeenBirth.cfm

46. Mincieli, L., Manlove, J., McGarrett, M., Moore, K., & Ryan, S. (2007). The relationship context of births outside of marriage: the rise of cohabitation. (Publication No. 2007-13). Washington, DC: Child Trends Research Briefs.

47. Albert, B. (2007). With one voice 2007: America's adults and teens sound off about teen pregnancy. Washington, DC: The National Campaign to Prevent Teen Pregnancy. Retrieved November 26, 2007, from http://www.thenational-campaign.org/resources/pdf/pubs/WOV2007_fulltext.pdf

48. The National Campaign to Prevent Teen Pregnancy. (2006). Science says: The public costs of teen childbearing. (Issue No. 30). Washington, DC: Author. Retrieved 11/23/2007 from http://www.thenationalcampaign.org/resources/pdf/SS/SS30_Costs.pdf

49. Davies, S., Dix, E. S., Rhodes, S. D., Harrington, K. F., Frison, S., & Willis, L. (2004). Attitudes of young African-American fathers toward early childbearing. American Journal of Health Behavior,28(5), 418-425.

50. Fagan, J., Bernd, E., & Whiteman, V. (2007). Adolescent fathers' parenting stress, social support, and involvement with infants. Journal of Research on Adolescence, 17(1), 1-22.

51. Hoffman, S. (2006). By the numbers: The public costs of teen childbearing. Washington DC: National Campaign to Prevent Teen Pregnancy.

52. MMWR Surveill Summ. (2004). STD-prevention counseling practices and human papillomavirus opinions among clinicians with adolescent patients - U.S., 2004. Washington, DC: Author.

53. Kirby, D. (2007). Emerging Answers 2007: Research Findings on Programs to Reduce Teen Pregnancy and Sexually Transmitted Diseases. Washington, DC: The National Campaign to Prevent Teen Pregnancy. Retrieved January 9, 2008, from http://www.thenationalcampaign.org/EA2007/EA2007_full.pdf

54. Centers for Disease Control and Prevention. (2007). STD Surveillance 2006. Washington, DC: Author. Retrieved December 10, 2007 from http://www.cdc.gov/std/stats06/default.htm

55. Fife, K., Fortenberry, J. D., Ofner, S., Katz, B. P., Morrow, R. A., & Orr, D. P. (2006). Incidence and prevalence of herpes simplex virus infections in adolescent women. Sexually Transmitted Diseases, 33(7), 441-444.

56. Department of Health and Human Services. (2007). HIV/AIDS surveillance report. Atlanta, GA: Centers for Disease Control and Prevention. Retrieved December 10, 2007 from http://www.cdc.gov/hiv/topics/surveillance/resources/reports/2005report/pdf/2005SurveillanceReport.pdf

57. Office On Women's Health. (2007, 11 December). Girls health: Symptoms of sexually transmitted diseases. Washington, DC: Author. Retrieved December 11, 2007, from http://www.girlshealth.gov/body/reproductive_health/rh.symptoms.cfm

58. Halpern-Felsher, B., Cornell, J. L., Kropp, R. Y., & Tschann, J. M. (2005). Oral versus vaginal sex among adolescents: perceptions, attitudes, and behavior. Pediatrics,115(4), 845-851.

59. Crosby, R., Salazar, L. F., DiClemente, R. J., Yarber, W. L., Caliendo, A. M., & Staples-Horne, M. (2005). Accounting for failures may improve precision: evidence supporting improved validity of self-reported condom use. Sexually Transmitted Diseases, 32(8), 513-515.

60. The National Campaign to Prevent Teen Pregnancy. (2007). Teen birth rate increase 2006: Some thoughts from the National Campaign to Prevent Teen and Unplanned Pregnancy. Washginton, DC: Author. Retrieved January 20, 2008, from http://www.thenationalcampaign.org/resources/pdf/NCHS_statement1.pdf

61. Ray, N. (2007). Lesbian, gay, bisexual and transgender youth: An epidemic of homelessness. Wahington DC: National Gay and Lesbian Task Force Policy Institute.

62. Herman-Giddens, M.E. (2006). Recent data on pubertal milestones in United States bhildren: the secular trend toward earlier development. International Journal of Andrology. 29(1), 241-246
Euling, S.Y., Herman-Giddens, M.E., Lee, P.A., Selevan, S.G., Juul, A., Sorensen, T.I.A., Dunkel, L., Himes, J.H. Telmann, G., & Swan, S.H. (2008). Examination of US Puberty-Timing Data from 1940 to 1994 for Secular Trends: Panel Findings. Pediatrics: 121, 172-191.

63. CDC. (December 2004). Vital and Health Statistics, Teenagers in the United States: Sexual Activity, Contraceptive Use, and Childbearing, 2002. 23, 24, 1-48 Retrieved February 1, 2009 from http:// www.cdc.gov/nchs/data/series/sr_23/sr23_024.pdf

64. CDC. (December 2004). Vital and Health Statistics, Teenagers in the United States: Sexual Activity, Contraceptive Use, and Childbearing, 2002. 23, 24, 1-48 Retrieved February 1, 2009 from http:// www.cdc.gov/nchs/data/series/sr_23/sr23_024.pdf

65. Gold, Melanie A., Sucato, Gina S., Conrad, Lee Ann E., & Adams, Paula J. (2004). Provision of Emergency Contraception to Adolescents. Journal of Adolescent Health, 35, 66-70.

66. Saewyc, E.M., Beringer, L.H., Blum, R.W., & Resnick, M.D. (1999). Sexual Intercourse, Abuse and Pregnancy Among Adolescent Women: Does Sexual Orientation Make a Difference? Family Planning Perspectives, 31(3): 127-131.

67. Saewyc, E.M., Beringer, L.H., Blum, R.W., & Resnick, M.D. (1999). Sexual Intercourse, Abuse and Pregnancy Among Adolescent Women: Does Sexual Orientation Make a Difference? Family Planning Perspectives, 31(3): 127-131.

68. STD Community Interventions Program (SCIP) (n.d.). Sexually Transmitted Diseases (STDs): What you need to know to stay healthy. Author, STD Control Branch, California Department of Health Services.

69. STD Community Interventions Program (SCIP) (n.d.). Sexually Transmitted Diseases (STDs): What you need to know to stay healthy. Author, STD Control Branch, California Department of Health Services.

70. Guttmacher Institute. (2007, August 1). State Policies in Brief: Minors' Rights as Parents. Retrieved February 1, 2009 from http://www.guttmacher.org/statecenter/spibs/spib_MRP.pdf.

71. Brein, M.J., & Willis, R.J., Costs and consequences for fathers, in Kids Having Kids: economic and social consequences of teen pregnancy, R.Maynard, Editor. 1997, The Urban Institute Press: Washington, DC. p. 95-143. As cited in: The National Campaign to Prevent Teen Pregnancy. "Why it Matters: Teen Pregnancy and Responsible Fatherhood." Retrieved from http://www.thenationalcampaign.org/why-it-matters/pdf/fatherhood.pdf

72. Hofferth, Sandra L., et al. (2001). The Effects of Early Childbearing On Schooling Over Time. Family Planning Perspectives, 33(6), 259–67.

73. Tan, Louisa H. & Julie A. Quinlivan. (2006). Domestic Violence, Single Parenthood, and Fathers in the Setting of Teenage Pregnancy. Journal of Adolescent Health, 38, 201–7.

74. Centers for Disease Control. "Condoms and STDs: Fact Sheet for Public Health Personnel." Retrieved February 6, 2009 from http://www.cdc.gov/condomeffectiveness/latex.htm

75. Oral Abstract D4a – Prevalence of Sexually Transmitted Infections and Bacterial Vaginosis among Female Adolescents in the United States: Data from the National Health and Nutritional Examination Survey (NHANES) 2003-2004. Retrieved from http://www.cdc.gov/stdconference/2008/media/summaries-11march2008.htm

76. Source: Centers for Disease Control. "Condoms and STDs: Fact Sheet for Public Health Personnel." Page last updated: February 6, 2009. http://www.cdc.gov/condomeffectiveness/latex.htm

77. Source: Centers for Disease Control. "Perspectives in Disease Prevention and Health Promotion Condoms for Prevention of Sexually Transmitted Diseases." MMWR Weekly. March 11, 1988 / 37(9); 133-7.
Retrieved from http://www.cdc.gov/mmwr/preview/mmwrhtml/00001053.html

78. Source: Centers for Disease Control. Fact Sheet. "Rumors, Myths and Hoaxes." Retrieved February 1, 2009 from http:///www.cdc.gov/hiv/resources/qa/hoax1.htm.